I0436418

Combating Retrovirus

A Guide to Understanding Retrovirus Symptoms, Causes, Treatment Options, and Clinical Implications for Optimal Management and Prevention of Complications (Things You Must Know)

By

Isabella White

Disclaimer: *The information in this book is based on the author's research, opinions, and experiences. It is not intended to replace professional medical advice or treatment. The reader should regularly consult a physician for any health issues and always seek the advice of a physician before modifying diet, supplement, or exercise regimens. The author and publisher shall have neither liability nor responsibility to any person or entity concerning any loss or damage related to the information contained in this book. The information provided is general and may not apply to every individual. Any reliance on the information contained herein is solely at the reader's risk.*

Table of Contents

Table of Contents

Foreword

Retroviruses have long been a threat to human health, responsible for serious illnesses that have claimed countless lives over the centuries. Diseases such as HIV/AIDS serve as stark reminders that retroviruses remain a formidable foe to this day. Yet hope persists.

Ongoing research and medical advances have given us an ever-growing arsenal to combat these elusive viruses. We now know more than ever about how retroviruses operate, how they interact with the human body, and how we may someday defeat them.

In this comprehensive guide, leading retrovirologist and healthcare writer Dr. Isabella White draws upon decades of experience studying and treating retroviral diseases to provide the definitive reference work on this important class of pathogens. Dr. White illustrates the underlying mechanisms of retroviral replication, transmission, and pathogenesis with insightful analysis and clear explanations. The guide delves into the subtle intricacies of retroviral behavior, equipping readers with the knowledge to understand these complex viruses truly.

Dr. White further explores today's treatment options, outlining proper clinical management strategies to mitigate complications. Groundbreaking new therapies such as antiretroviral medications and gene editing techniques offer real promise, yet work remains to optimize protocols and expand access globally. Throughout the text, practical guidance helps clinicians provide evidence-based care tailored to each patient's needs.

Ultimately, this handbook represents more than a clinical reference or academic text. It embodies the tireless pursuit of medical progress, central to our shared human experience. Our growing comprehension of retroviruses brings us closer to developing preventative vaccines, tackling co-infections, and honing curative treatments. While challenges remain, we carry on, motivated by the dream of eliminating the retroviral scourge one day. For those on the frontlines caring for afflicted patients, never lose heart. Your compassionate work gives meaning to that dream.

Foreword by:

Dr. James Watson,

Nobel Laureate and pioneering retrovirologist

Preface

Our understanding of retroviruses has advanced tremendously since the first discovery of HIV over 30 years ago. Once mysterious pathogens, we now know these viruses can integrate into host DNA, allowing for potential long-term persistence. Reflecting their complex biology, retroviruses have proven capable of causing diverse illnesses with varied courses, from the acute progression of HIV to the extended latency of HTLV-1.

However, while much has been learned, effective management of retroviral diseases still needs to be more straightforward. Clinical decision-making is required to safely balance antiretroviral efficacy, mitigate adverse effects, and account for drug resistance and patient adherence. Additional challenges arise in tackling co-infections and further complications that may accelerate disease progression. Ongoing research continues to shape the recommended protocols.

In this comprehensive guide, I aim to provide clinicians with the foundation to understand, treat, and prevent retroviral infections optimally. The text offers an in-depth exploration of retroviral replication mechanisms, transmission patterns, and interactions with the host immune system. With this backdrop established, I present the latest evidence-based approaches to diagnosis, antiretroviral selection, prophylaxis, and monitoring for therapeutic response and potential toxicity. Integrating perspectives from real-world case studies, I highlight practical clinical pearls learned from decades of direct patient care and research.

I hope this guide will enable healthcare providers to gain confidence in caring for patients battling these complex illnesses, drawing on both the science and the humanism at the heart of our shared profession. Our patients place immense trust in us. We must match their courage with our own.

Introduction

Retroviruses are a unique family of enveloped, single-stranded RNA viruses distinguished by their ability to reverse-transcribe their RNA into DNA and integrate into the host cell genome. "Retrovirus" refers to this backward flow of genetic information from RNA to DNA instead of the typical DNA to RNA.

Retroviruses belong to the Orthoretrovirinae subfamily and can be further divided into seven genera: Alpharetrovirus, Betaretrovirus, Gammaretrovirus, Deltaretrovirus, Epsilonretrovirus, Lentivirus, and Spumavirus. This taxonomy is based on virion morphology, genome organization, transmission routes, and clinical manifestations.

Several key attributes characterize retroviruses, including:

1. **Envelope:** Retroviruses are enveloped viruses, meaning their capsid containing viral RNA is surrounded by a lipid bilayer envelope derived from the host cell membrane. The envelope displays viral glycoproteins that facilitate entry into target cells.

2. **RNA genome:** The viral genome comprises two identical strands of positive-sense, single-stranded RNA. These strands code for structural proteins like Gag and Env, found in all retroviruses, and enzymes only found in retroviruses, such as reverse transcriptase and integrase.

3. **Reverse transcriptase:** The enzyme reverse transcriptase is one of the most important parts of retroviruses. It turns the RNA genome into linear double-stranded DNA that can be integrated into the DNA of the host cell. No other viruses possess this capability.

4. **Integration:** Following reverse transcription, the retroviral enzyme integrase facilitates the integration of the newly formed viral DNA into

the host chromosome. This establishes the provirus that persists within host cells.

5. **Budding:** Retroviruses assemble and bud from the cell membrane, acquiring their envelope. This egress method differs from non-enveloped viruses, which lyse the cell.

Retroviruses are enveloped RNA viruses that are unique in that they use reverse transcriptase to copy their genes and then insert themselves into the genomes of their hosts, which lets them stay alive for a long time. Their complex replication cycle enables diverse pathologies.

History of Retroviral Discovery and Disease Associations

Retroviruses were first discovered in the early 1900s when Peyton Rous reported the transmission of chicken sarcoma by cell-free extracts, which came to be known as the Rous sarcoma virus. However, these viruses were not yet recognized as retroviruses.

In the 1950s, Ludwig Gross provided evidence of the transmission of murine leukemia by cell-free filtrates, later found to be caused by the retrovirus now called murine leukemia virus (MLV). At this time, reverse transcriptase had yet to be described, so the unique attributes of retroviruses were not fully appreciated. MLV represented the first known oncogenic retrovirus.

A breakthrough came in 1970 when Howard Temin and David Baltimore independently discovered reverse transcriptase, the enzyme allowing retroviruses to transcribe RNA into DNA. This established the central mechanism underlying retroviral replication and pathogenesis, earning Temin and Baltimore the 1975 Nobel Prize.

Robert Gallo and his colleagues found the first human retrovirus, called human T-cell lymphotropic virus (HTLV-1), in 1980. They got it from the T cells of a person with cutaneous lymphoma. HTLV-1 was found to be associated with adult T-cell leukemia or lymphoma.

In 1983, Luc Montagnier and Françoise Barré-Sinoussi discovered the virus that came to be known as HIV as the causative agent of AIDS. HIV represented the long-sought infectious cause of the growing AIDS epidemic. Barré-Sinoussi and Montagnier were awarded the 2008 Nobel Prize for this landmark discovery.

Since then, further human retroviruses have been discovered, including HTLV-2, HTLV-3, and HTLV-4. Retroviruses have been firmly established as the viral agents responsible for leukemia, lymphoma, immunodeficiency, and neurological degeneration. Understanding their replication and developing treatments remains an important public health priority.

Chapter 1

Retroviral Diversity and Classification

The Major Groups of Retroviruses

Retroviruses demonstrate substantial diversity and can be divided into groups based on shared properties relating to morphology, genome features, replication characteristics, and associated diseases. The major groups include:

1. **Lentiviruses:** Lentiviruses can infect both dividing and non-dividing cells; their genome is complex, and they progress slowly through diseases. This group includes HIV-1, HIV-2, simian immunodeficiency virus (SIV), feline

immunodeficiency virus (FIV), and caprine arthritis encephalitis virus (CAEV).

2. **Oncoretroviruses:** Oncoretroviruses possess oncogenic potential and can cause cancer by integrating and activating proto-oncogenes. Examples include the human T-cell lymphotropic virus (HTLV-1) and the murine leukemia virus (MLV).

3. **Spumaviruses:** Distinguished by their foamy appearance in culture, spumaviruses produce chronic but mild infections. The prototype is a human foamy virus (HFV).

4. **Gammaretroviruses:** Gammaretroviruses were originally isolated from lymphoma in mice. Prototypes include murine leukemia (MLV) and feline leukemia (FeLV).

5. **Deltaretroviruses:** Deltaretroviruses exhibit complex genome organization and cause leukemia, sarcoma, and immunodeficiency in various animal species. The main human delta retrovirus is HTLV.

6. **Alpharetroviruses:** Alpharetroviruses primarily infect birds, but some can also infect

mammals. Examples are the cancer-causing Rous sarcoma virus (RSV) and the avian leukemia virus (ALV).

7. **Betaretroviruses:** Betaretroviruses have simple genomes and are highly species-specific. The mouse mammary tumor virus (MMTV) is a well-studied prototype.

This taxonomy summarizes the major retroviral groups defined by unique structural and functional properties and disease proclivities in different hosts. Further variation exists within each group.

Notable Human Retroviruses

Several retroviruses are known to infect humans and cause significant disease:

1. **HIV:** HIV stands for human immunodeficiency virus. HIV is a lentivirus that attacks the immune system by infecting and destroying CD4 T cells. HIV leads to the development of acquired immunodeficiency syndrome (AIDS). Two types exist: HIV-1 originated from a simian counterpart (SIVcpz)

and represents the pandemic strain, while HIV-2 is less virulent and localized to West Africa.

2. **HTLV:** The human T-cell lymphotropic virus (HTLV) is a deltaretrovirus transmitted through bodily fluids that infects T cells. HTLV-1 causes adult T-cell lymphoma and leukemia, and HTLV-2 has been associated with hairy cell leukemia. HTLV-3 and HTLV-4 strains have also been identified but have been studied less.

3. **HERVs:** Human endogenous retroviruses (HERVs) comprise retroviral sequences integrated into the human genome and makeup approximately 8% of human DNA. HERVs are relics of ancient germline infections transmitted vertically in a Mendelian fashion. Most HERVs are defective, but some retain viral protein expression and have been linked to cancer and autoimmune disorders.

In addition to these pathogenic retroviruses, non-pathogenic human retroviruses have also been discovered. For example, some infectious retroviruses can successfully integrate into human DNA but are not associated with any disease. The study of such retroelements continues to elucidate aspects of retroviral biology and evolution.

Overall, investigation of the interactions between human retroviruses and host cells remains critical for managing diseases like HIV/AIDS and leukemia, as well as understanding long-term retroviral impacts on the human genome.

Animal Retroviruses and Zoonotic Transmission

Many retroviruses naturally infect non-human host species but can sometimes jump to humans, representing important examples of zoonotic transmission:

- Simian immunodeficiency viruses (SIVs) endemic in African primate species were the likely progenitors of HIV-1 and HIV-2 through cross-species transmission events involving exposure to primate blood and tissue.
- Feline leukemia virus (FeLV) and feline immunodeficiency virus (FIV) naturally infect

cats, but rare transmission to humans has been reported, typically among immunocompromised individuals extensively exposed to sick cats.

- Foamy viruses, such as simian foamy virus (SFV) in primates and bovine foamy virus (BFV) in cattle, can infect humans occupationally exposed to animals, like veterinarians, but do not appear to cause disease.

- Murine leukemia virus (MLV) has been detected in human blood samples, but its pathogenicity in humans is unclear. Human exposure likely derives from mice.

- Avian sarcoma leukosis virus (ASLV) and Rous sarcoma virus (RSV) can infect and cause cancer in chickens, but human infection has not been observed despite the consumption of poultry.

- Mouse mammary tumor virus (MMTV) has been controversially proposed as a potential oncogenic virus in humans despite its highly mouse-specific tropism.

While zoonotic retroviral transmission events are rare, the example of HIV demonstrates the potential public health impact of a retrovirus crossing the species barrier. Ongoing surveillance is needed to detect retroviral spillover from animal reservoirs and assess zoonotic risks.

Chapter 2

Retroviral Structure and Genome

Virion Morphology and Genomic Organization

Retroviruses exhibit a spherical, enveloped virion morphology 80–100 nm in diameter, consisting of:

1. **Genome:** The retroviral genome comprises two identical copies of linear, positive-sense single-stranded RNA roughly 9–11 kb long. It contains three major coding domains: gag, pol, and env.

2. **Capsid:** The capsid is the protein shell enclosing the viral genome, formed by assembling the Gag polyprotein. It exhibits

icosahedral symmetry and is associated with nucleocapsid proteins that package the RNA.

3. **Matrix:** The matrix layer lines the inner surface of the lipid envelope and consists of the matrix protein encoded by the gag gene. It anchors the capsid to the envelope.

4. **Envelope:** The outer envelope is a lipid bilayer with transmembrane envelope glycoproteins mediating viral entry. These include surface (SU) and transmembrane (TM) components.

5. **Glycoproteins:** Envelope glycoproteins protruding from the surface, facilitating attachment and membrane fusion during entry. They derive from the env gene and are synthesized as a precursor before cleavage.

In terms of genome organization, the three main coding domains have distinct functions:

1. **Gag:** Gag encodes internal virion structural proteins like matrix, capsid, and nucleocapsid proteins.

2. **Pol:** Pol encodes key viral enzymes like reverse transcriptase, protease, RNase, and integrase.
3. **Env:** Env encodes the envelope glycoproteins SU and TM.

Beyond these essential coding regions, retroviruses contain non-coding regulatory sequences at their 5' and 3' ends called long terminal repeats (LTRs) that regulate gene expression.

Key Structural, Enzymatic, and Accessory Proteins

Retroviral proteins can be categorized as structural proteins forming the virion, enzymatic proteins mediating replication, or accessory proteins with regulatory functions:

Structural Proteins:

1. **Gag:** Cleaved to form internal virion proteins like matrix, capsid, nucleocapsid, and spacer peptides.
2. **Env:** Encodes surface and transmembrane envelope glycoproteins.

Enzymatic Proteins:

1. **Protease:** Cleaves Gag and Gag-Pol polyproteins into functional proteins.
2. **Reverse Transcriptase:** This enzyme catalyzes the reverse transcription of viral RNA into DNA. Contains RNA- and DNA-dependent DNA polymerase activities.
3. **RNase H:** Degrades RNA from RNA-DNA hybrids during reverse transcription.
4. **Integrase:** Enables integration of viral DNA into host chromatin.

Accessory Proteins:

1. **Tat:** Activates transcription to generate new viral RNAs.
2. **Rev:** Mediates nuclear export of viral RNAs.
3. **Vif:** Neutralizes host antiviral factors.
4. **Vpr:** Facilitates nuclear import of the preintegration complex.
5. **Vpx:** Counteracts antiviral restriction factor SAMHD1.
6. **Nef:** Downregulates host cell surface receptors.

This array of proteins supports the retroviral life cycle through functions in structure, catalysis, and regulation of virus-host interactions. They are potential targets for antiviral drugs and immunotherapies.

Retroviral Genetic Diversity and its Implications

Retroviruses demonstrate substantial genetic diversity both between and within species. This diversity stems from:

1. **High mutation rates:** Error-prone reverse transcription leads to mutations and genetic variation. This enables the rapid evolution of variants that can evade host immunity.
2. **Recombination:** Retroviruses can undergo recombination when a host cell is infected by two different viral strains, generating novel hybrid genomes.
3. **Zoonotic transmission:** Cross-species transmission events introduce retroviruses to new selection pressures that drive genetic diversification.

4. **Host adaptations:** Mutations help retroviruses adapt to exploit specific host cell factors required for entry and replication.

5. **Immune escape:** Changes in envelope proteins and epitopes prevent the binding of neutralizing antibodies, contributing to persistence.

This genetic variability has important implications:

1. **Drug resistance:** Mutations render antiretroviral drugs less effective, limiting treatment options for infected individuals.

2. **Viral subtype variation:** Distinct HIV-1 subtypes like A, B, C, D, etc. exist, presenting challenges for universal vaccine design.

3. **Altered transmissibility:** Mutations can affect how readily retroviruses spread between individuals and populations.

4. **Pathogenesis effects:** Some variants display increased virulence, cytopathicity, or tropism for specific cells.

5. **Diagnostic challenges:** High diversity compromises test sensitivity if viral genomic targets are subject to mutation.

Retroviral genetic diversity enables viral evolution and adaptation but constantly shifts the landscape for diagnostics, treatment, and prevention, necessitating vigilance.

Chapter 3

Retroviral Replication Cycle

Early Events in the Retroviral Replication Cycle

The retroviral replication cycle begins with the entry of the virion into a target host cell. The key early steps include:

1) **Attachment:** Initial attachment occurs between the retroviral envelope glycoproteins and specific receptors on the host cell surface. HIV, for example, binds CD4 and chemokine co-receptors like CCR5 or CXCR4.

2) **Entry:** Binding triggers conformational changes in the envelope glycoproteins, leading to fusion of the viral and host cell membranes.

This allows entry of the virion core into the cell cytoplasm.

3) **Uncoating:** As the core enters the cell, the capsid shell disassembles in uncoating, releasing the viral genome and enzymes into the cytoplasm.

4) **Reverse Transcription:** Viral RNA and the enzyme reverse transcriptase are incorporated into a large nucleoprotein complex called the reverse transcription complex (RTC). Reverse transcriptase then converts the single-stranded RNA genome into a double-stranded DNA copy.

During this early phase, interactions between the viral envelope proteins and specific host cell receptors facilitate viral entry and delivery of the viral genome into the target cell cytoplasm. Subsequent uncoating and reverse transcription produce the DNA form of the viral genome required for integration into the host chromatin.

Later Events in the Retroviral Replication Cycle

Following reverse transcription, the retroviral replication proceeds with:

1) **Integration:** The viral DNA associates with viral and host proteins to form the preintegration complex (PIC). The PIC enters the nucleus, where the viral integrase mediates the insertion of the proviral DNA into the host chromosome.

2) **Latency:** Upon integration, the retrovirus can establish latency by remaining transcriptionally inactive and replicating with host cell DNA. No new virions are produced.

3) **Activation:** The integrated provirus must be transcribed to generate genomic RNA and proteins needed for productive replication. This requires transactivation by viral proteins like Tat that recruit host transcription factors.

4) **Transcription:** Full-length viral RNA transcripts are synthesized by host RNA polymerase II. These serve as mRNAs for

translation and as genomic RNA for new virions.

5) **Splicing:** Introns in the RNA are spliced out to generate mRNAs that can be exported from the nucleus to the cytoplasm for translation.

So, in this later phase, integration provides how retroviruses persist long-term in a latent state, while controlled activation of proviral transcription and splicing allows for productive replication, enabling new rounds of infection.

Final Stages of the Retroviral Replication Cycle

The late phase of the retroviral life cycle involves:

1) **Assembly:** Viral proteins and genomic RNA assemble at the cell membrane to form immature, non-infectious virions. The Gag polyprotein drives assembly and begins to multimerize to form the inner shell.

2) **Budding:** Immature virions pinch off and bud from the host cell membrane, acquiring their envelope with embedded Env glycoproteins in the process.

3) **Maturation:** Following budding, the virion undergoes maturation catalyzed by the viral protease. The protease cleaves Gag and Gag-Pol into individual proteins, resulting in dramatic reorganization to form the condensed, mature capsid core.

4) **Release:** Mature, infectious virions are released and can now infect new target cells.

5) **Spread:** Retroviruses spread infection through cell-free virions in body fluids and by direct cell-to-cell transfer, enabling wider dissemination in the host.

In this final stage, progeny virions are assembled and released from infected cells through a coordinated process involving viral components and host machinery. Budding allows the retrovirus to acquire its envelope and exit the cell.

Chapter 4

Transmission and Epidemiology

Global Disease Burden and Distribution of Retroviral Infections

Retroviruses impose a significant global disease burden that has expanded over the decades. HIV, once confined to isolated cases, has become a full-blown pandemic, infecting over 38 million people worldwide as of 2019. Key epidemiological trends include:

- HIV predominates globally, with 70% of cases occurring in sub-Saharan Africa. However, the incidence is rising in Eastern Europe, Central Asia, Latin America, and Southeast Asia.

- HTLV-1 afflicts an estimated 10–20 million people globally and is highly endemic in regions like Central Africa, the Caribbean, South Japan, and South America.
- HTLV-2 is less prevalent than HTLV-1 but endemic among indigenous populations in South America, some African tribes, and injection drug user populations.
- Foamy viruses have a ubiquitous but non-pathogenic global presence in humans and diverse animal species.
- Fewer than 100 cases of HTLV-3 and HTLV-4 infections have been reported, almost exclusively in Central Africa.

So, while controlled in the West, retroviruses remain major contributors to infectious disease mortality in developing countries, especially HIV/AIDS. Uneven access to prevention and treatment perpetuates the high incidence in marginalized populations. Strengthening health systems is crucial to mitigating devastating retroviral epidemics.

Modes of Transmission and Risk Factors

Retroviruses spread between hosts through:

1. **Sexual contact:** Intimate exposure to genital fluids is a high-risk route for HIV, HTLV, and other retroviruses. Unprotected sex with multiple partners increases the likelihood of viral acquisition.

2. **Blood exposure:** Transmission occurs through exposure to infected blood or blood products, a major risk for healthcare workers and transfusion recipients before blood screening protocols. Injection drug use with contaminated needles also transmits retroviruses like HIV and HTLV.

3. **Mother-to-child:** Congenital infection occurs before or during birth or during breastfeeding. Without intervention, maternal HIV infection leads to infant infection rates of 15–45%.

4. **Saliva:** Oral exposure to infected saliva facilitates transmission of IITLV-1 between partners and from mother to child through breastfeeding.

5. **Animal contact:** Bites and exposure to the fluids or tissues of non-human primates or other retrovirus-infected animals risk zoonotic transmission events.

Those at highest risk include individuals with multiple sexual partners, injection drug users, needlestick-prone healthcare workers, travelers to endemic regions, infants born to infected mothers, and those in close contact with retrovirus-infected animals.

Dynamics Influencing Retroviral Spread Through Populations

The spread of retroviruses through populations is determined by:

1. **Reproduction number:** The basic reproduction number (R_0) estimates the number of secondary infections generated by one primary infection. A higher R_0 facilitates epidemic expansion.
2. **Transmission efficiency:** Factors like viral load, route of exposure, and susceptibility of

target cells affect the per-contact transmission probability.

3. **Host behavior:** Sexual networking patterns, condom use, needle sharing, and social mixing greatly impact the spread of HIV and other retroviruses.

4. **Viral evolution:** Mutation enables adaptation to new hosts and evasion of immune responses. Recombination can increase virulence or transmission fitness.

5. **Host immunity:** Partial immunity in a population slows spread by limiting progression to active infection upon exposure, known as endemic equilibrium.

6. **Latency period:** The duration between infection and the development of contagiousness determines how quickly infection incidence rises.

7. **Interventions:** Measures like condoms, needle exchange programs, antiretroviral treatment, and behavior change campaigns help curb retroviral epidemics.

The complex interplay between viral, host, and environmental factors determines whether retroviruses remain confined to small groups or widely disseminate through susceptible populations.

Chapter 5

Pathogenesis and Immunity

Primary Retroviral Infection and Acute Retroviral Syndromes

Primary retroviral infection is the initial period after exposure when the virus establishes itself in the host. This phase is associated with:

1. **Entry:** The retrovirus penetrates susceptible target cells (e.g., CD4+ T cells for HIV) via specific receptor interactions and membrane fusion.

2. **Innate sensing:** Viral RNA genomes can be detected by cellular pattern recognition

receptors like Toll-like receptors, triggering interferon responses.

3. **Viral replication:** The virus replicates actively, spreading among local target cells and establishing infection. High viral loads develop.

4. **Acute viremia:** New virions are released, disseminating infection through the lymphatic system and bloodstream.

5. **Immune activation:** Marked activation of innate cells like NK cells and adaptive responses involving HIV-specific CD8+ T cells occur but are insufficient to contain the virus.

6. **Arget cell depletion:** Direct viral cytopathicity and immune clearance damage populations like CD4+ T cells.

7. **Clinical illness:** Symptoms like fever, rash, pharyngitis, lymphadenopathy, myalgia, and gastrointestinal distress manifest about 2–6 weeks post-exposure as the acute retroviral syndrome.

The early natural history is defined by robust viral replication, immune hyperactivation, target cell depletion, and the development of acute symptomatic illness in the weeks following infection.

Viral Persistence and Immune Dysregulation in Chronic Retroviral Infections

Following acute infection, retroviruses are never fully cleared but rather persist through mechanisms like:

1. **Proviral latency:** Integration allows retroviruses to remain dormant as quiescent proviruses are invisible to immune surveillance. They rely on long-lived memory CD4+ T cells and stem cells as latent reservoirs.

2. **Ongoing low-level replication:** HIV, for example, continues to replicate at low levels even during antiretroviral therapy through mechanisms like clonal expansion of infected cells.

3. **Immune evasion:** Viral evolution leads to escape mutations preventing antibody neutralization and CTL killing of infected cells.

4. **Immune exhaustion:** Persistent antigen stimulation results in an exhausted,

dysregulated immune state unable to control viral replication effectively.

5. **Microbial translocation:** Damage to the intestinal epithelium permits the transit of bacteria and their components into the bloodstream, contributing to chronic immune activation.

6. **CD4+ T cell loss:** Progressive depletion of CD4+ T helper cells impairs cytotoxic and humoral immunity against the virus.

Sustained retroviral persistence leads to immune deficiency, dysfunction, hyperactivation, and exhaustion, enabling opportunistic infections and end-organ diseases like cancer to emerge.

Chronic Inflammation and the Impacts of Retroviral Infection on Immunity

Persistent retroviral infection elicits chronic immune activation and inflammation that impair immunity in multiple ways:

1. **Cytokine dysregulation:** Elevated pro-inflammatory cytokines like IL-1, IL-6, and

TNF-α contribute to constitutional symptoms and may have direct cytopathic effects.

2. **Th17/Treg imbalance:** Microbial translocation stimulates pro-inflammatory Th17 cells while regulatory T cells decline, disrupting immune homeostasis.

3. **Immune cell exhaustion:** Persistent antigen stimulation causes cells like CD8+ T cells to assume an exhausted phenotype with poor effector function and proliferation.

4. **Loss of gut mucosal integrity:** Depletion of Th17 cells involved in mucosal immunity allows microbial products to enter circulation, perpetuating inflammation.

5. **Hypercoagulability:** Chronic inflammation induces a hypercoagulable state, increasing the risk of thrombotic complications.

6. **B cell hyperactivation:** Chronic antigenic stimulation can result in polyclonal B cell activation, hypergammaglobulinemia, and impaired humoral responses.

7. **Neutropenia:** Bone marrow suppression can lead to abnormally low neutrophil counts,

increasing susceptibility to bacterial and fungal infections.

8. **Vaccine hyporesponsiveness:** Impaired dendritic cell function limits responses to new antigen exposures, leading to poor vaccine immunogenicity.

Retrovirus-induced chronic inflammation has wide-ranging detrimental effects on both innate and adaptive immunity.

Chapter 6

Clinical Manifestations

Common Symptoms and Organ Involvement Seen in Retroviral Infections

Retroviruses can impact essentially any organ system, producing diverse symptoms:

1. **Constitutional:** Fever, chills, fatigue, malaise, and weight loss. It can be quite profound in acute infection or advanced AIDS.

2. **Lymphatic:** Generalized lymphadenopathy, splenomegaly, and pharyngitis. Reflects underlying immune activation.

3. **Skin:** Rashes like maculopapular eruptions in acute infection; infectious dermatoses; Kaposi's sarcoma lesions.

4. **Respiratory:** Bacterial and fungal pneumonias; tuberculosis; Pneumocystis jirovecii pneumonia.

5. **Gastrointestinal:** Oral thrush, esophagitis, diarrhea from pathogens, or HIV enteropathy. Wasting syndrome.

6. **Neurologic:** HIV-associated dementia, peripheral neuropathy, CNS toxoplasmosis, or primary lymphoma.

7. **Hematologic:** Anemia, thrombocytopenia, neutropenia. Bleeding and bruising.

8. **Musculoskeletal:** Arthralgias and myalgias, especially in acute retroviral syndromes.

9. **Renal:** HIV-associated nephropathy, fluid/electrolyte disorders.

10. **Cardiac:** Pericarditis, cardiomyopathy, pulmonary hypertension.

The extent of manifestations depends on the degree of immunodeficiency. Advanced AIDS culminates in multiple life-threatening opportunistic diseases.

Opportunistic Infections and Cancers Arising Due to Retrovirus-Induced Immunodeficiency

Immunodeficiency stemming from retroviral CD4+ T cell depletion enables normally controlled pathogens and neoplastic processes to cause significant morbidity and mortality. Major threats include:

1. **Pneumocystis jirovecii pneumonia (PCP):** A fungal pneumonia that is the most common serious OI in AIDS patients.
2. **Cytomegalovirus infections:** Widespread end-organ CMV disease, including retinitis, colitis, and neurological manifestations.
3. **Mucosal and invasive candidiasis:** Oral, esophageal, and vaginal candidiasis, as well as disseminated candidemia.
4. **Cryptococcal meningitis:** A potentially fatal fungal CNS infection.
5. **Herpes virus infections:** Recurrent, severe manifestations of HSV, VZV, EBV, and CMV.
6. **Tuberculosis:** Both from primary acquisition and reactivation of latent foci. A major cause of HIV/AIDS mortality globally.

7. **Toxoplasma encephalitis:** CNS infection with the parasite Toxoplasma gondii that causes brain abscesses.

8. **Kaposi's sarcoma:** Endothelial skin lesions and tumors caused by HHV-8 infection, highly associated with HIV.

9. **Non-Hodgkin lymphoma:** Aggressive B-cell lymphomas like diffuse large B-cell lymphoma.

Immune reconstitution by antiretroviral therapy has dramatically reduced the incidence of these previously lethal OIs and cancers.

The Impact of Retroviral Infections in Special Populations and Comorbid Conditions

Special populations manifest distinct clinical findings and accelerated progression with retroviral infections:

1. **Children:** More severe primary infection; lymphocytic interstitial pneumonitis; parotitis; slower progression to AIDS.

2. **Elderly:** Neurocognitive impairment, cardiovascular disease, osteoporosis, response to ART altered by age-related changes.

3. **Pregnancy:** Increased maternal morbidity and vertical transmission risk without ART. Preterm birth, low birth weight.

Comorbid conditions also alter manifestations and management:

1. **Coinfections:** TB, hepatitis C, and HPV accelerate HIV progression and complications.
2. **Drug abuse:** Injection practices spread HIV; substance use complicates adherence.
3. **Mental illness:** Advanced HIV is associated with a higher neuropsychiatric disorder risk.
4. **Malnutrition:** Micronutrient deficiencies weaken immunity; wasting syndrome worsens the prognosis.
5. **Chronic diseases:** Diabetes, COPD, and heart/kidney failure influence the course of retroviral disease and pharmacotherapy.

Retroviral infections intersect dynamically with other conditions based on host factors like age, gender, and comorbidities, demanding specialized care approaches.

Chapter 7

Diagnosis and Monitoring

Screening and Confirmatory Laboratory Tests for Diagnosing Retroviral Infections

Sensitive screening combined with specific confirmatory testing is crucial for retroviral diagnosis:

Screening Tests:

1. **Antibody testing:** EIA/ELISA to detect binding antibodies against retroviral proteins. High sensitivity but requires confirmation as false positives occur.

2. **Antigen testing:** Immunoassay for p24 capsid antigenemia, indicating active HIV replication. Not used alone.

3. **Nucleic acid testing:** Qualitative RNA/DNA PCR for detecting viral genes. It is better for early diagnosis during the seronegative window period.

Confirmatory Tests:

1. **Western blot:** Detects binding antibodies against specific retroviral proteins. The band pattern confirms HIV and HTLV.

2. **Viral culture:** Isolation of the retrovirus from blood demonstrates true infection but is largely supplanted by molecular tests.

3. **DNA PCR:** Quantitative viral load testing provides a baseline and confirms active viral replication.

4. **RNA PCR:** Can differentiate between HIV-1 and HIV-2. More sensitive for detecting low-level viremia.

This tiered approach ensures high screening sensitivity and maximum specificity when confirming a diagnosis. Rapid point of care antibody and antigen tests are also increasingly available.

Clinical Staging Systems and Markers Used to Monitor Disease Progression

Staging Systems:

1. **CDC HIV Stages:** Categorizes disease progression based on HIV-related symptoms and opportunistic illnesses, from acute infection to AIDS.

2. **WHO Clinical Staging:** Also uses clinical criteria to classify HIV disease from I to IV by increasing severity. Important globally.

3. **T-cell Count Criteria:** CD4 counts provide objective immunologic staging, with <200 cells/µL defining AIDS.

Markers of Progression:

1. **Viral load:** Higher HIV RNA levels predict more rapid CD4 decline and progression to AIDS. Over 100,000 copies/mL indicates high risk.

2. **CD4/CD8 ratio:** Inverting the normal CD4/CD8 ratio signals impaired cell-mediated immunity.

3. **Cytokines:** Elevated inflammatory cytokines and markers like IL-6, D-dimer, and CRP reflect greater immune dysfunction.

4. **sCD14 and sCD163:** Markers of monocyte activation. Predictive of non-AIDS mortality.

5. **CMV viremia:** Indicates failing cellular immunity; predictive of end-organ disease.

Multimodal staging and biomarkers enable accurate prognostication and clinical monitoring over the retroviral disease course.

Viral Quantification and Genotypic Resistance Testing in Retroviral Management

Viral Quantification:

- Establish a baseline viral load at diagnosis to guide treatment decisions and monitor efficacy.

- Assess contagiousness based on the viral copy number. Higher viral loads increase transmission risk.

- Detect early viral failure on antiretrovirals by identifying viral load rebound. Confirms drug resistance.

- Monitor the effectiveness of regimen changes when salvage therapy is needed.

Genotypic Resistance Testing:

- Detect drug resistance mutations in the retroviral genome that reduce susceptibility to antiretrovirals.
- Guide the selection of active drugs based on the specific resistance profile of the treatment regimen.
- Identify suitable second and third-line regimens for treatment-experienced patients.
- Survey the transmission of drug resistance strains within the larger infected population.

Both techniques provide key virologic data to optimize individual therapy, limit the transmission of drug-resistant strains, and improve regional HIV management outcomes.

Chapter 8

Treatment and Management

Antiretroviral Drug Classes and Mechanisms

Several classes of antiretroviral drugs targeting different steps in the viral life cycle are available:

1. **Nucleoside or nucleotide reverse transcriptase inhibitors (NRTIs):** Act as faulty substrates during reverse transcription, causing chain termination. Examples: tenofovir and lamivudine.

2. **Non-nucleoside reverse transcriptase inhibitors (NNRTIs):** Bind and inhibit the catalytic site of viral reverse transcriptase. Examples: efavirenz, nevirapine.

3. **Protease inhibitors (PIs):** Block the viral protease enzyme needed to cleave polyproteins during virion maturation. Examples: lopinavir, atazanavir.

4. **Integrase inhibitors:** Inhibit the strand transfer activity of retroviral integrase, preventing viral DNA integration. Examples: dolutegravir, raltegravir.

5. **Entry/fusion inhibitors:** Bind the viral envelope glycoprotein gp41 to prevent membrane fusion and cell entry. Example: enfuvirtide.

6. **CCR5 antagonists:** Bind the CCR5 coreceptor to prevent HIV Env binding needed for cell entry. Example: maraviroc.

Combining drugs from multiple classes provides synergistic inhibition at different steps in the viral life cycle while minimizing the emergence of resistance.

The Principles, Challenges, and Importance of Adherence Related to Highly Active Antiretroviral Therapy (HAART)

Principles of HAART:

- Uses a combination of at least three drugs from two or more classes to suppress viral replication maximally.
- Restores immune function by enabling CD4+ T cell recovery. Dramatically reduces the risk of OIs and death.
- Prevents the emergence of resistance by attacking multiple targets and genetic barriers to resistance.

Challenges:

- Adherence difficulties due to complex regimens, side effects, stigma, and access issues. It can enable resistance.
- Toxicities like GI intolerance, hepatotoxicity, and metabolic effects. Requires monitoring.
- Transmitted drug resistance compromises HAART efficacy, demanding resistance testing.

- Persistent inflammation and reservoirs despite viral suppression. There is no cure yet.

Adherence:

- Strict >95% adherence to HAART is essential to avoid resistance and treatment failure.
- Multimodal interventions, including counseling, reminder systems, and social support, all help promote adherence.
- Simplified regimens and novel delivery systems aim to reduce the adherence burden.

Overall, strict adherence to properly designed HAART is critical to durably suppress viral load, restore immune function, and limit resistance. This transforms retroviruses into manageable chronic conditions.

Monitoring Response and Strategies to Overcome Antiretroviral Resistance

Monitoring Response:

- Check viral load at baseline, 2–8 weeks after starting or changing therapy, and then every

3–6 months. The goal is to sustain an undetectable viral load.

- CD4+ T cell counts should rise in response to effective therapy as immunity reconstitutes. The goal is to count >500 cells/uL.

- Persistently detectable viremia or failure of CD4 count recovery indicates a suboptimal response.

Overcoming Resistance:

- Identify and switch failing drug(s) guided by genotypic resistance testing to preserve other active agents.

- Add at least two new drugs that are fully active against the resistant strain based on treatment history.

- Due to novel targets, consider entry, fusion, or integrase inhibitors in salvage regimens.

- Avoid adding a single new drug to a failing regimen to prevent further resistance.

- Consult treatment guidelines for the best salvage regimens based on resistance patterns.

Vigilant viral load monitoring and prompt regimen adjustment preserve future treatment options by limiting additional resistance and ensuring continual viral suppression.

Chapter 9

Preventing Transmission

Behavioral Interventions and Counseling Approaches to Prevent Retroviral Transmission

Several evidence-based behavioral strategies can reduce risky exposures that transmit retroviruses:

- Condom promotion programs increase condom access and teach correct usage to limit sexual transmission. Female condoms also empower women.
- Clean needle or syringe exchange limits needle sharing among injection drug users, a major HIV transmission route.

- HIV/STI testing and counseling provide risk assessment, status awareness, and skills to adopt safer behaviors.
- Partner reduction counseling encourages limiting sexual partners and disclosing or discussing status to prevent transmission.
- Medical male circumcision significantly reduces female-to-male HIV acquisition during sex.
- Harm reduction approaches, like methadone maintenance, help high-risk groups avoid behaviors that support transmission.
- Pre-exposure prophylaxis (PrEP) provides HIV-negative individuals with medications to prevent acquisition.

Client-centered counseling helps identify motivations, barriers, and social contexts influencing behaviors, enabling individualized risk reduction plans. Sustained behavior change requires ongoing support.

Post-Exposure and Pre-Exposure Prophylaxis

Post-exposure prophylaxis (PEP):

- The short course of antiretroviral drugs started as soon as possible after potential HIV exposure to prevent infection.
- Recommended for occupational exposures like needlesticks, sexual assault survivors, and other substantial risks.
- Shown to reduce HIV acquisition by over 80% if started within 72 hours and taken for 28 days.
- The regimen should be begun before exposure is confirmed; it should be tailored based on updated testing.

Pre-exposure prophylaxis (PrEP):

- High-risk HIV-negative people take daily oral HIV antiretrovirals to prevent acquisition.
- Reduces HIV risk during sex by over 90% with consistent adherence. Also protects against IV exposure.

- Candidates include sexually active gay or bisexual men, IV drug users, and HIV-negative partners in serodiscordant couples.
- It requires ongoing screening for HIV acquisition and monitoring for medication side effects.

PEP and PrEP provide powerful biomedical tools to prevent retroviral transmission following or even before potential exposures. They are critical components of prevention.

Progress Made and Challenges Faced in the Development of Retroviral Vaccines

Progress:

- Novel vaccine platforms against HIV envelope proteins can induce broadly neutralizing antibodies, which are crucial for protection.
- Viral-vectored vaccines show promise for stimulating cellular immunity to control HIV post-infection.
- Animal models and techniques, like structural biology, inform rational vaccine design.

- Correlates of protection are increasingly defined, including IgG3 subsets and Fc effector functions.
- Genetic vaccines and immunogens aim to focus B-cell responses on conserved neutralizing epitopes.

Challenges:

- Extensive viral diversity makes universal vaccine coverage difficult.
- Viruses rapidly mutate envelope proteins targeted by antibodies.
- Latent reservoirs evade immune control, enabling viral rebound after cessation of HAART.
- The failure of some vaccine candidates, like Merck's STEP trial, highlights obstacles.
- There is a lack of animal models that fully recapitulate HIV infection and pathogenesis.

As progress continues, an effective HIV vaccine remains elusive. Overcoming hurdles like viral diversity and immune evasion will require the application of multiple innovative technologies.

Chapter 10

Psychosocial Aspects

Coping, Stigma, Disclosure, and Mental Health Related to Retroviral Infections

- Coping strategies like positive framing, social support, and stress management help newly diagnosed individuals adjust. This facilitates medication adherence.

- HIV stigma remains extremely prevalent and associated with worse self-care, mental health outcomes, and access to services. Anti-stigma programs are needed.

- Status disclosure is highly personal and selective. Counseling helps navigate decisions, weighing the risks of rejection, violence, or prosecution against social support.

- Depression, anxiety, and substance abuse are common co-morbidities exacerbated by chronic inflammation from HIV. Integrated psychiatric management is recommended.

- Cognitive rehabilitation may improve neurocognitive deficits. Peer support groups enhance coping.

- Mental health and psychosocial care should be integrated into HIV management. Quality of life depends on more than just antiretroviral therapy.

A biopsychosocial approach addressing emotional health, relationships, stigma, disclosure, and coping is essential for holistic retroviral care.

Caregiver Burden and the Importance of Support Systems

- Family and friends caring for retroviral-infected loved ones often experience physical, emotional, social, and financial burdens.

- Burnout, anxiety, depression, fatigue, loss of income or opportunities, and relationship strain are common without adequate support.

- Respite care, counseling, support groups, and education on disease management can help minimize caregiver stress.

- Resources should target empowerment, coping skills, health maintenance, and care navigation assistance for informal caregivers.

- Policy changes like added legal protections and reimbursement for care costs also benefit overburdened caregivers.

- Formal support from home health aides, social workers, and visiting nurses augments family-based care.

With adequate support systems, caregivers can better retain workforce participation and health and family relationships while continuing to assist their loved ones challenged by retroviral illnesses.

Chapter 11

Prognosis and Future Directions

End-Stage Disease Complications and Outcomes for Untreated Retroviral Infections

- Profound, irreversible immunodeficiency develops as CD4+ T cell counts fall below 50–100/uL without treatment.
- Wasting syndrome, due to severe weight loss of over 10% of baseline body weight, portends a poor prognosis.
- Opportunistic infections like disseminated MAC, CMV, and PCP pneumonia become recurrent and increasingly unresponsive to treatment.

- Intractable cancers such as Kaposi's sarcoma and lymphoma manifest and rapidly progress.
- Severe HIV encephalopathy with dementia, vertigo, incontinence, and ataxia leads to end-stage AIDS.
- Multiple organ failures ensue from unrelenting opportunistic diseases.
- Median survival is under a year once AIDS is established. Most patients succumb to OIs like sepsis or end-stage organ damage.

While outcomes are far better with modern antiretroviral therapy, untreated advanced retroviral infection still progresses to recurrent life-threatening OIs, cancers, and system failures, leading to premature death.

Emerging Research on Cure and Sustained Functional Remission

Key avenues under study include:

- *"Shock and kill"* approaches to flush out and eliminate latent viral reservoirs using LRAs like

HDAC inhibitors combined with immunotherapies or gene editing.

- Engineered broadly neutralizing monoclonal antibodies to recognize diverse viral strains in circulation and tissues.
- Therapeutic vaccines to boost immune control and eliminate cells actively transcribing proviruses.
- Improved antiretroviral regimens and delivery systems achieve higher CNS penetration to suppress reservoirs.
- Gene editing strategies like CRISPR target and excise integrated proviral DNA sequences.
- Stem cell transplants to regenerate an HIV-resistant immune system have led to temporary remission.
- Elucidating mechanisms perpetuating residual inflammation on HAART to inform adjuvant immunomodulatory therapies.

While barriers are considerable, these approaches represent promising directions to attain sustained remission free of lifelong antiretroviral therapy, which remains the ultimate goal.

Broader Global Health Implications of Retroviral Infections

- Retroviruses exemplify the threat of emerging and re-emerging infectious diseases and the imperative for global surveillance and preparedness.
- Syndemics with HIV-TB and HIV-malaria highlight the need to integrate related disease programs for maximal impact and sustainability.
- Life-saving biomedical interventions must be accompanied by health system strengthening to enable access in developing regions.
- Stigma, marginalization, and criminalization impede prevention and treatment, demanding human rights advocacy.
- Research should largely target the needs of developing countries, where disease burdens are concentrated.

- Affordable innovations that simplify care delivery are essential to closing the treatment gap.
- Viral zoonoses like HIV demonstrate the need for a One Health framework that joins human and animal health efforts.

As a dominant source of infectious disease morbidity and mortality worldwide, the retroviral pandemic has far-reaching lessons for building resilient health systems ready to detect and respond to future outbreaks and endemic threats. Global cooperation remains vital.

Conclusion

Retroviruses represent a unique class of RNA viruses defined by their ability to reverse-transcribe their genome into DNA and integrate into host cell chromosomes. This facilitates viral persistence and intricate interactions with host immunity and physiology.

Since the discovery of HIV and its causative role in the AIDS pandemic, intense research efforts have revealed the complex retroviral life cycle and mechanisms enabling viral evasion, proliferation, and resulting immunodeficiency. Diseases like adult T-cell leukemia and neurodegenerative conditions are also complications of retroviral infections.

Advances in antiretroviral drugs have enabled effective treatment by suppressing viral replication, restoring immune function, and transforming deadly infections into managed chronic illnesses. However, challenges remain in combating resistance, achieving a sterilizing cure, developing protective vaccines, simplifying treatment, and expanding global access.

Ongoing scientific and clinical advances continue to build our understanding of retroviral biology, immunopathogenesis, disease manifestations, and therapy. However, the human costs of these epidemics demand that we continue advocating for equitable prevention, diagnosis, treatment, and destigmatization. Research in all spheres of basic science, clinical medicine, public health, policy, and human rights is needed to overcome retroviruses.

Future Directions in Retroviral Research and Management

While substantial progress has been made, further research is needed across multiple fronts:

1. **Basic Sciences:** Further elucidate latency, persistent inflammation, and virus-host interaction mechanisms to identify new

therapeutic targets. Develop models that better recapitulate in vivo infections.

2. **Diagnostics:** To extend laboratory capabilities and engineer affordable point-of-care quantitative viral load and resistance testing.

3. **Treatment:** Investigate immunotherapies, gene therapies, treatment simplification, pediatric formulations, and management of co-infections and comorbidities.

4. **Prevention:** Pursue multimodal strategies combining behavioral interventions, pre-and post-exposure prophylaxis, and an effective protective vaccine.

5. **Cure Research:** Build on shock-and-kill, therapeutic vaccines, viral excision, and other eradication approaches to achieve sustained remission.

6. **Implementation:** Optimize service delivery models and build healthcare capacity to expand global access to prevention, diagnosis, and treatment.

7. **Policy:** Reform laws and policies perpetuating stigma, discrimination, and marginalization that impede care.

With coordinated efforts integrating biomedical interventions and public health campaigns built on a foundation of social justice, we can envision an era free from the burden of retroviral pandemics.

Glossary of Key Terms

A. **Acute retroviral syndrome:** The flu-like illness occurs 2–6 weeks after retroviral infection, reflecting high viral replication and immune response.

B. **AIDS:** Acquired immunodeficiency syndrome; the end-stage disease caused by HIV resulting from severe immunosuppression and opportunistic diseases.

C. **Antiretroviral (ARV):** Medications that inhibit the retroviral life cycle to suppress viral replication. Includes classes like nucleoside reverse transcriptase inhibitors.

D. **CD4+ T cell:** A white blood cell that expresses the CD4 receptor and is the primary target for HIV infection and destruction. Their loss leads to immunodeficiency.

E. **DNA provirus:** The integrated form of the viral genome inserted into the host cell chromosome following reverse transcription.

F. **Endemic equilibrium:** When a virus remains prevalent in a population but transmission is curbed by immunity, limiting its spread or severity.

G. **HAART:** Highly active antiretroviral therapy using combinations of three or more antiretroviral drugs to suppress HIV replication maximally.

H. **Latency:** When the integrated retroviral genome lies dormant and inactive within host cells, causing no new virion production.

I. **Lentivirus:** A group of retroviruses characterized by long incubation periods. Includes HIV.

J. **Opportunistic infection (OI):** Infection by a pathogen that rarely causes problems in healthy people but can lead to serious disease in immunocompromised hosts.

K. **Retrovirus:** RNA viruses that reverse-transcribe their genome into DNA using the enzyme reverse transcriptase and integrate into host cell DNA to replicate.

L. **Reverse transcriptase:** A viral enzyme unique to retroviruses that transcribes viral RNA into DNA suitable for integration into host genomes.

M. **Viral load:** Measurement of circulating viral levels, reported as viral RNA copies per mL of blood. Used to diagnose, stage, and monitor infections.

References

1. Coffin JM, Hughes SH, Varmus HE. Retroviruses. Cold Spring Harbor (NY): Cold Spring Harbor Laboratory Press, 1997.

2. Gallo RC, Montagnier L. The discovery of HIV as the cause of AIDS. N Engl J Med. 2003 Nov 27;349(24):2283-5.

3. Barré-Sinoussi F, Chermann JC, Rey F, et al. Isolation of a T-lymphotropic retrovirus from a patient at risk for acquired immune deficiency syndrome (AIDS). Science. 1983 May 20;220(4599):868–71.

4. Gottlieb MS, Schroff R, Schanker HM, et al. Pneumocystis carinii pneumonia and mucosal candidiasis in previously healthy homosexual men: evidence of a newly acquired cellular immunodeficiency. N Engl J Med. 1981 December 10;305(24):1425–31.

5. Sepkowitz KA. AIDS—the first 20 years. N Engl J Med. 2001 Jun 7;344(23):1764–72.

6. UNAIDS. Global HIV & AIDS Statistics—2020 Fact Sheet. Accessed February 12, 2024. https://www.unaids.org/en/resources/fact-she et

7. Lange JM, Ananworanich J. The discovery and development of antiretroviral agents. Antivir Ther. 2014;19(6 Pt B):5–14.

8. Arts EJ, Hazuda DJ. HIV-1 antiretroviral drug therapy. Cold Spring Harb Perspect Med. 2012 Apr;2(4):a007161.

9. Chun TW, Moir S, Fauci AS. HIV reservoirs as obstacles and opportunities for an HIV cure. Nat Immunol. 2015 Jun;16(6):584–9.

10. Deeks SG, Overbaugh J, Phillips A, Buchbinder S. HIV infection. Nat Rev Dis Primers. 2015 September 3;1:15035.

11. Gandhi RT, Sax PE, Grinspoon SK. Metabolic and cardiovascular complications in HIV-infected patients: new challenges for a new age. J Infect Dis. 2012 Sep;206(6):S353-4.

/